Essential Tips for Beginning Martial Artists 2

By Pat Smith

I0419866

My first booklet, *Essential Tips for Beginning Martial Artists*, was very popular, so I decided it might be helpful to continue the theme with a second volume.

I find that prospective martial arts students, and new students, are often misled by poor and misguided advice. I think those of you who are new to the martial arts, or who would like to get started, and even some of you who may be more seasoned martial artists, will benefit greatly from the simple and practical advice that I provide in these booklets.

My hope is that these tips, as with those of my previous booklet, will help you avoid many of the mistakes that I made when just starting the martial arts, and even, in some cases, years later.

Now, I did not make all of the mistakes that I mention. For example, I've never practiced or trained with sharp weapons. But I know of other students of the martial arts who have and who regretted their mistakes later. I will say that I anticipate some of my advice will anger many of the martial arts instructors out there, especially those who sell lots of videos and books. The reason is because so much of the martial arts has become commercialized for profit. I understand this, to a degree.

Martial arts instructors, particularly those who are full-time, have to make money; it's a business. But some of them are clearly trying to get rich on the martial arts, and they cut corners and don't warn their customers. There's nothing wrong with buying martial arts products (books, videos, etc.), but I want you to understand some of the risks involved, and get to know the limits of the products you use, so you can know how best to use them. So, without further ado, here are 14 important basic tips, building on the tips from the first booklet, that will help you get the most out of your martial arts training and practice.

Tip #1:
Do NOT Learn Martial Arts
from Books

This should be a no-brainer, but I can't tell you how many students have approached me after attempting to "learn" martial arts from books. Some martial arts instructors even try to teach whole martial arts systems, or large parts of them, through books!

Often this is a money-making scheme, because they know there is a market out there for would-be martial artists that either don't have the discipline to spend the time it takes to really learn a martial art, or else they don't have the money, or, for whatever reason, they are too frightened or too embarrassed to begin a martial art from the ground up.

Many people are embarrassed to be beginners. You have to lose this fear, or at least move beyond it, or else you will never succeed in martial arts training. The best masters I know still consider themselves beginners, in some way. As they move forward, as they climb one mountain peak in their martial arts accomplishments, they recognize further peaks off in the distance. You have to start somewhere, and that somewhere is always at the beginning.

Typically ranked with a white belt. Don't be embarrassed by the white belt. It's not a badge of honor, but that's not what it's about.

I cannot emphasize this strongly enough: ***<u>DO NOT TRY TO LEARN MARTIAL ARTS FROM A BOOK!!!</u>*** This is particularly true of complicated kata or forms work, either empty hand or with weapons. The more complicated the form, the more complicated the weapon, the more you are almost assured of missing the essential subtleties.

This is probably most true of the Chinese martial arts, and especially of the northern styles. But it remains true of all martial arts. Bruce Lee had a popular set of volumes on exercises and self-defense techniques, and I knew a number of people who would read those books, and then try to learn from them how to perform the techniques.

One of them was a street fighter who wanted to implement them, not for self-defense, but for fighting prowess in his school and neighborhood. He had some real street fighting experience, as had the others whom he fought. But, unlike them, he had no training whatsoever. He tried to learn all sorts of techniques—like finger jabs—but when he fought others who had boxed or had wrestled, they tore him apart. He ended up in the hospital, but was fortunate not to have been killed or imprisoned. He made a lot of mistakes, including going against my very first "tip" or advice from my last booklet—don't pursue the martial arts if your goal is to hurt others.

The point is that there absolutely no substitutes for an actual living instructor. Books cannot replace an instructor. You cannot learn the martial arts from a book. So why should you read my blog posts and booklets, and any other material I might produce? That brings us to the next tip.

Tip #2:
How to Use
Martial Arts Books
for All They Are Worth

You can profit from martial arts literature, if you use it wisely. How? What benefit can books, articles, blogs, etc., on the martial arts be if you can't learn a martial art, or self-defense techniques from them?

The truth is that if the martial arts literature is good, you can learn about martial arts history, the particular distinctive characteristics, etc., of the styles about which you're reading.

You can also learn good training advice, or even self-defense advice, if the author is knowledgeable and reliable. Right there those are some huge benefits of reading about the martial arts that should not be underestimated.

The problem is that such reading is far too often overestimated. Reading about martial arts has some very real limits, and you need to be well aware of those limits if you don't want to end up getting yourself killed, going to prison, or getting injured.

Let's face it, in the world we live in today, you will always run the risk of death and injury, and perhaps imprisonment. If you practice the martial arts, risk of injury comes with the territory. I've never met a martial artist who has escaped bruises, for example, in their training. The point is you want to decrease your chances of sustaining injuries, and trying to learn a martial art from a book only increases your chances.

There are other ways that martial arts literature can be beneficial to you. But I should warn you up front, that these ways are more for advanced students and masters than for novices.

The newer you are to the martial arts, the less you'll be able to benefit from martial arts literature beyond the general information I mentioned above.

If you are more seasoned, if you know what to look for, you can learn about some of the subtleties like hand position, foot position (is the heel supposed to be up, is your front foot on your toes, should your foot be flat on the ground, etc.), arm angle, etc.

These subtleties are not trivial, by any stretch of the imagination. Such subtleties differentiate the true masters from those who don't really know what they're doing. And the difference can be seen and felt.

Even the novice can often tell the difference from a true master performing a technique or a kata/form from someone with significantly less skill. The difference is that the novice might not know what was different in the details. They might say, "the master performed with more power," or just "the master's performance looked better."

The differences might actually have been in posture, and footwork, in synchronizing hand and foot techniques and weapons, or in the angles of blocks and strikes, and the twisting of the waist.

The ways that books are best used are by those who already know the style. If you already know the style, the books can serve as reminders, or even help give you further insights. The better you know the style or the technique, the more you'll be able to benefit from the books.

Tip #3:
Do NOT Learn
Martial Arts
from Videos

This advice is very similar to that above concerning books. The difference is, with free online videos like Youtube, more would be martial artists—especially teenagers and young adults—are trying to learn martial arts and self-defense techniques from videos, especially online.

There have been whole martial arts video markets for a very long time. Just open up any martial arts magazine, and you'll likely find video offers to learn complete styles. There are entire websites devoted to teaching the martial arts remotely online through video.

Now, to be fair, some of these programs are better than others. I do not claim to have first-hand knowledge of all of these programs. In fact, I confess that I've never used any of these programs. I've always sought out instructors to teach me the martial arts. But you should be clear that videos are no substitute for an actual instructor.

That being said, some of these programs are obviously better than others.

The better ones, though, especially the ones geared toward self-defense, are, in my mind, perhaps some of the most dangerous, because they give you a sense of achievement and confidence that might prove deadly on the street.

I have seen some samples of these on Youtube, and I've also read the descriptions of some of the online programs, and have spoken with many "students" of such video material. So, here are some things to consider about the various video options out there. Some of these programs are just videos. You watch the techniques, you hit pause, you try to imitate what you saw, etc. Some will show the techniques from different angles.

Other programs will offer you a form of belt or rank "testing," where you video yourself performing what you've "learned" from their videos, and, for a fee, can submit your video to the instructor for them to evaluate. I have never heard of anyone doing this and NOT getting promoted.

To be fair, this is all coming from anecdotal evidence. There may be loads of exceptions out there that I'm just not aware of. A response might be to point out that something similar happens at some martial arts schools.

I'm aware that some martial arts schools exist where students typically don't fail their rank exams. This is not necessarily a mark against those schools, however. The reason I say that is because any instructor that is any good at teaching martial arts will recommend a student postpone a test if they don't think the student is ready yet. They should have a fairly accurate gauge of this from observing the student in class and from speaking with any other instructors the school might be using.

This is more difficult with the larger schools, but it shouldn't be overly difficult. It's not like the students have to be perfect. I've never witnessed a black belt exam where those who earned the black belts performed perfectly. In fact, in an ideal black belt exam, the chief instructor would provide individual feedback making some corrections to help the newly minted black belt go even further.

At the same time, there are some schools that have "guaranteed" black belt programs, etc., where no one ever fails, and some of the students certainly should have failed. I'd be wary of any school that guarantees a black belt, especially those programs that advertise, "Black Belt in One

Year." I'd stay away from any school like that.

Some of the more technologically sophisticated programs now have online teaching where you can purchase video lessons online. You can watch videos for rank, or for special topics (e.g., knife self-defense). You can also Skype (or some equivalent) with instructors to get advice and feedback.

Sometimes they may even be able to schedule appointments to watch you perform the techniques and provide feedback. These will obviously be better programs than the earlier ones I mentioned. I've seen these programs for some Japanese and Chinese styles.

Regardless of the style you're interested in, the quality of your "training," if we can call it that, from such programs will be dependent upon numerous factors, especially the following:

1) your ability to translate what you see on video to what you are practicing in real life. This is not that simple, since on the video their techniques will look as though they're being performed on the opposite side of you. What's to your right on the video will be their left. This is not easy, even though the same is often true in regular class instruction.

2) the technology and your use of it. The more ability the instructor on the other end has to observe and correct your techniques the better.

3) your instructor's ability to observe over video. Whether you're sending in a video of yourself practicing, or it's live, the instructor at the other end needs to be able to pick up on the subtleties of your mistakes. I would imagine that this is very difficult, except for big mistakes.

4) the amount of time and quality of your own practice apart from video "training sessions."

5) the actual abilities of your instructor in the martial arts he or she is teaching.

6) the actual abilities of your instructor to teach.

7) the diversity of angles, of repetition, and quality of verbal instruction, on the video.

This is no small task. I would highly recommend against anyone trying to learn a martial art from video, even from these more technologically savvy online programs. I'll say it again: there's absolutely no substitute for a real live instructor that is with you. An instructor who can feel your technique, and who can let you feel their technique. A lot of martial arts learning has to do with "feeling":

feeling a technique preformed on you as well as feeling how the technique is performed on others.

Tip #4:
How to Use
Martial Arts Videos
for All They Are Worth

Does this mean that you should completely stay away from martial arts videos? Absolutely not! In fact, I'll be posting some videos from Youtube to my martial arts blog regularly.

The important thing is to use such videos wisely and in ways that are most beneficial. Videos are superior to books for seeing techniques, forms/kata practice, etc.

You can watch someone perform the technique, which is much easier than looking at pictures in a book or reading the descriptions.

I still recommend against this approach to learning the martial arts, because in learning the martial arts, you need to do more than "see" a performance.

You NEED appropriate and helpful **_CORRECTION_**_!!!_ Even in the old days of Chinese martial arts, where a sifu might perform a technique or a form one time, and expect the student to be able to imitate what was demonstrated, the sifu would correct the student, sometimes quite severely. Correction is essential. It's very hard to do this well over video. Perhaps some of these online programs are better than the old days of VHS mail away martial arts programs, but I remain skeptical—but open to correction!

As with books, the best way to use such videos is as reminders of what you've already learned. Maybe you know that a particular kata or a specific technique is going to be required on an upcoming exam. You know the kata, or the technique, but you want to watch others perform it. It can be great to watch some Youtube videos of masters performing the same kata or technique.

Although, be forewarned, unless it's your own instructor giving the example of how he or she wants the kata or technique performed on the exam, the video you see might be different than what is expected of you.

Sometimes there is a variety of ways the kata are performed by different masters, or by different schools that use the same kata. This is notorious in the Chinese martial arts, and I've observed this especially with the Northern Praying Mantis Kung Fu forms I know.

When it comes to techniques the degrees of varying can be equally great. Several of them might be effective, but on exams you typically have to perform them a specific way. There are exceptions to this (like Aikido black belt tests which often permit more variety, or any style that requires full-contact fighting for an exam).

Videos can be great to refresh your memory, but be careful. Always listen to your own instructor over the video and be aware that differences might exist. Not every "master" on Youtube is a real master. People make mistakes, etc.

You can also learn a lot of good information and pick up helpful tips and advice on martial arts videos. This is especially true if you already have familiarity with the techniques. The instructor might want to emphasize a subtlety that you're somewhat familiar with but haven't paid sufficient attention to, but you may already know the basic technique, may have even passed it on an exam.

Videos can be very helpful here if it's from a good instructor. I don't recommend videos for beginners, just because they can often cause more harm than good. As you advance, they can be helpful along the lines I mentioned above. And, if you have a lot of money, some of those online programs might be a great supplement to actual live instruction.

Tip #5:
Listen to Your Body

Physical and mental toughness can be a great asset in the martial arts, as in life, but you really want to learn to listen to your body. Obviously you want self-defense training to mimic a real situation as much as possible while keeping yourself and your training partner as safe as possible.

But you simply can't treat training and practice sessions like hand-to-hand combat in the middle of a battle in a war. Obviously, if you're a member of an elite forces unit and you've lost your explosives are gone, and your gun is out of ammo, and the enemy is at your throat, you have no choice, you have to fight through whatever harm comes to your body, as best as you can, or you might die.

If your fingers break from a strike, you trip and twist your knee out of joint, your enemy stabs a sharp object through your rib cage collapsing a lung . . . you're not going to call a time out and get medical attention. Your very survival will depend on your fighting through the pain and damage in a situation that is beyond less than ideal.

But you can't treat training and practice sessions like that. You have to rest. You have to take care of injuries. Now you don't want to stop and take time out for every bruise you get. You might have to in the case of bloody noses, or any blood, so as not to damage the mat or carpet, and so as to prevent the spread of diseases and illnesses.

But if you think you injured your knee, or sprained an ankle, or broke a bone, stop practicing! Take a break. Seek medical attention, and then find out how best to heal. You might have to take some time off practice, or at least practice less intensely.

You have to learn "good" pain from "bad" pain. What I mean by that is there's a difference between the soreness of a muscle that has worked out intensely and is growing stronger from the soreness of a pulled muscle or the pain of a strain.

If you've never practiced a martial art before, the chances are, your muscles will be sore for at least the first few weeks of practice. If the martial art involves lots of kicks, punches, low stances, or throws, your soreness might be pretty severe at first. If you're sore, don't stop training or practicing! Don't injure yourself, but if it's simply muscle soreness from use, you don't want to take a full week off or longer, because it will only take more time for your body to become accustomed to the activity. Take a day off, maybe two, but the quicker you can get back to training and practice, the quicker your sore muscles will become accustomed to the activity.

This is not the case with an injury. If you're injured, you may have to take off a few weeks, or even more time, depending on the severity of the injury and where you were injured. Always check with your physician about an injury, how to treat your injury, and when to get back to training.

General rule of thumb, listen to your body. Don't do what your body is not comfortable doing. If you can't take a break fall, let your instructor know, and skip that activity.

Sometimes, in martial arts like Aikido where there are quite a few techniques performed on the knees, older practitioners or those with knee injuries cannot safely perform those techniques. You might want to ask your instructor about trying to just do those techniques from a standing position---- although, of course, suwari waza (performed from on one's knees) techniques in Aikido should actually make the toes more sore than the knees if done correctly.

In some instances, you might have to switch martial arts styles. Aikido and some of the Chinese Internal arts like Tai Chi and Hsing-I, might be more suited to practitioners with lots of injuries or infirmity from old age. Aikido can be quite vigorous, but in my experience, instructors are usually pretty flexible with the abilities of students with injuries, and if the techniques are performed correctly, they don't take any physical strength—the caveat here is that it often takes years of practice to get to that point.

Beginners notoriously muscle through Aikido techniques. Part of the reason for this is that Aikido uses your opponent's force against them. If you're a beginner, then the partner, the uke, is probably going to attack slowly, so as not to hurt you. But, in slow attacks, there's not much force to speak of, so you have to muscle through more than you would were they going at full speed.

At the same time, often the older and physically weaker Aikido students learn to perform the techniques properly quicker than the stronger and younger students, because they have to. So old age, physical weakness, and related infirmities can sometimes be a real strength for the study of Aikido. Bottom line: listen to your body.

Tip #6:
Never Practice/Train
with Sharp Weapons

This tip should also be a no-brainer, as should virtually all of the advice I've been giving in these first two booklets. Unfortunately, this advice is not always heeded. Students want to give a sense of reality to their training and practice.

No matter how good you are, if you use a sharp weapon, chances are you're going to get cut. With the popularity of sharpened traditional Asian swords for collectors, some companies have increasingly been selling these weapons for that purpose, and usually with the appropriate warnings.

The problem I've noticed is that they include words and phrases in their advertisements that often "encourage" their potential buyers, albeit not always explicitly, that these weapons can be used for personal defense, sometimes against home invasion, other times against would be attackers.

If you have the money and the interest, you can now buy traditional Chinese broadswords and butterfly swords that are combat ready, so sharp they could hack an opponent in half, and even fell trees.

Let's face it, men seem to be hard-wired to like sharp objects. I'm sure some women do to, but I don't know many boys who aren't fascinated by knives. The same goes for guns of course. Would a Chinese broadsword make a good home defense weapon? I don't know. There might not be much space to wield it, depending on your home.

But as someone who has made the mistake of practicing my Kung Fu broadsword forms inside (with wooden and unsharpened metal swords), I can tell you that lots of walls and furniture (and the ceiling) can get damaged very easily. It would be horrible (albeit perhaps humorous from a distance) to pull out your broadsword when the invader enters, only to get it stuck in the cabinet as you attempt to swing it near the invader, who might pull out a gun and end the whole thing right there.

Note: Chinese broadswords are typically a hacking sword that uses your shoulder more than writs or elbows, and thus, unlike some other Asian swords, require extended arms and a bit of space to use properly.

And can you imagine carrying around a sharpened Japanese sword on the street?!?! That's not even legal in Japan anymore, and hasn't been for over a hundred years—since 1876 to be precise. As cool as it sounds, such "self-defense" weapons are not very practical. Knives are another story, but I plan on an entire booklet devoted to knives, as well as many blogposts, so I'll leave that topic alone for the moment.

Regardless of the possible uses of sharp weapons for self-defense and defense against home invasion, they are a firm NO when it comes to training and practice. There's no better way to injure yourself and others than use a sharp blade in practice. Whether it's a sword form or practicing knife self-defense, sharp weapons spell blood, injury, and perhaps death.

I know countless martial artists, including some top masters, who have had the misfortune of having to defend themselves on the street against knife-wielding assailants. All of them have been cut and have the scars to prove it. If you're up against a knife, a razor blade, or another sharp instrument, you're probably going to get cut. End of story.

The same is true with training. I remember my first knife self-defense training, and we were using very flexible rubber knives. We had been practicing techniques for over a year. When it came to training, the opponent tried to mimic a real knife attack, full-contact. The defender was limited in that we couldn't perform the techniques full-contact because the potential damage was much worse than that of the rubber knife.

I had many years of martial arts training under my belt, and I don't think the fake blade of that knife missed me for a single technique. It "cut" my fingers, my hands, my neck, my arms, my leg, etc. My chest and ribs were thoroughly bruised after that training session. It taught me a good lesson, though: if I'm on the street, and that had been for real, I might be dead, and I certainly would have been cut.

Had we been using a real blade, I would have been taken to the hospital, or the morgue. Never ever train with sharp weapons. And, what's more, in the case of knife-self defense, unless you are using very stylized techniques, the kind that won't likely be used against you on the street but may help you learn defenses that can be applied against real attacks, make sure to wear protective gear for your eyes, no matter how soft the fake knife may be.

Tip #7:
Use Padded Weapons
or
Head Protection
as Appropriate

This advice goes for hard flexible weapons, like nunchaku, 3 section staff, 2 section staff, etc. If you're practicing the nunchaku, I would advise using the foam padded ones that are sold to kids before moving on to hard wood, or whatever you will eventually train with.

My preferred nunchaku for practice are hard wood connected by rope. Nunchaku practice can be a great forearm and shoulder workout. But if you get hit in the head at full speed with hard nunchaku, you can knock yourself out. So, to avoid brain damage, start with padded nunchaku.

The same goes for the various section staffs, most famously the 3 section staff of Kung Fu (both southern and northern styles use this staff). It's a very powerful and elegant weapon, in fact, one of my favorites. It's incredibly difficult to learn, despite videos and books that are sold regularly trying to teach this weapon.

When I began the martial arts, if you wanted to study the 3 section staff, you had to get the real thing. Perhaps there were padded ones around, but I never heard of them nor ever saw any. Now, inexpensive padded 3 section staffs can be purchased easily online and shipped to your door.

I will give one warning, and it's less an issue for nunchaku than the 3 section staff. This is the warning, that unlike nunchaku, because of the weight of the 3 section staff, a much lighter padded one may not adequately prepare you for practicing with the real thing. With the nunchaku, this is not the case, in my experience.

Despite the weight difference, perhaps because the handles are so small with nunchaku, compared to the 3 section staff, foam padded can be very good training for the real ones. With the 3 section staff, you might want to consider getting head gear or even a football helmet. Trust me, you don't want to hit yourself in the head with a real 3 section staff!!!

And one of the trickier aspects to the staff is that the faster it's moving, the safer you are—so long as you are doing the technique correctly. The slower it's moving, the more likely you are to hit yourself in the head, the groin, and in the face (all of which

I've done to myself . . . and take my word for it, it's not fun).

Tip #8:
Do Not Rush Rank Promotion

Ranking in the martial arts is rather a silly affair. Yes, it's good to keep children motivated, and for some reason, Americans (and I'm an American) tend to be focused on rank—"You do martial arts? Are you a black belt?" How many times have you heard or asked this question?

I never ask someone their rank. I do, on occasion, ask how long they've been training and practicing the martial arts. That will tell you far more than rank ever will. Aikido tends to be one of those martial arts that is closest to the original tradition of not ranking with belts. In traditional Aikido there's just the white belt and the black belt. Sure, there's still the 5 kyu's of the white belt, and 10 dan's of the black belt. If you're a black belt or higher you get to wear the hakama, which looks a little like a dress, but which can hide your footwork.

Rank is not that important. Now, of course, please celebrate exuberantly your children who progress in rank. That's great! In fact, I think you should go out and celebrate when you pass exams and move up in rank. That's great too! Just remember, though, that rank is not the same as ability, although ideally there is some correspondence.

The important thing is not that you advance rank as fast as possible, but rather that you learn the material and hone your skills as much as possible. One of the most important determining factors in your acquisition of true skill in the martial arts—beside receiving helpful corrections from your instructors—will be practice, practice, practice. Putting in hours of practice outside of formal classes (training). The repetitions will be key.

Don't worry about rank as much as skill. There are no short cuts to acquiring skill. It will take a lot of sweat, probably some tears, and possibly some blood (hopefully not too much of the latter).

Finally, always check with your instructor to see if he or she thinks you're ready to advance before taking a test. No need to waste money on a test you're not ready for.

At the same time, don't ever be discouraged by failing a test that you prepared for. That's difficult, even near impossible, especially when you have to pay for the test anyway.

But, and I don't know to emphasize this enough, you can learn a lot and grow a ton from failing a test. Failed tests are not necessarily failure, then can be very much a productive part of the learning process and of the process of gaining necessary skills and eventually achieving martial arts mastery.

If you really prepared hard for an exam, and your instructor thought you were ready, but when it came time for it, you couldn't quite perform, it probably had more to do with nerves—or poor judgment on the instructor's part—than anything else.

If your style or school requires full-contact fighting, or any sparring at all as part of the test, then it could also have to do with the other opponent. Either way, don't worry about it. Keep practicing, look at the failure itself as an achievement, and try again next time. It may not require working harder, it just might be a matter of more repetition in practice.

For those who often test at the earliest possible time, over the years, I think they find that they tend to know the techniques just enough to pass them on the test, but really get them down cold later.

Tip #9:
Do Not Rush
Learning New Techniques—
Quality Over Quantity

Students, especially young students and new students (regardless of age) often want to learn lots of new techniques every class or lesson. This is a mistake.

Some schools cater to this, and I think that too is a mistake, but sometimes for financial reasons, instructors are left with little choice.

You have to work for quality over quantity. What good is practicing 100 different techniques against a shoulder grab followed by face punch, if you're practiced those many techniques only a few times?

If you're out and about and in that situation, chances are you won't be able to use any of those techniques. Much better to master one technique against such a situation, and to have practiced it ten thousand times. Repetition is key.

On the street, if you are in a violent encounter, you won't likely have a lot of time to think. You will most likely react. In such a scenario, if you use any martial arts at all, you will use what comes to you naturally and instantly. Those, if anything at all, will likely be the simplest techniques, the ones you have practiced the most. And if you don't have thousands of repetition under your belt, than you probably won't "naturally" react with a martial arts technique at all, because you haven't yet developed sufficient muscle memory to deal with the situation which will unfold at near lighting speed.

Be patient, and work on one technique, not many. A few techniques should be fine. If you're practicing Karate or Kung Fu, then in an hour's class, in addition to warm ups, one kick, one empty hand technique, and some portion of a kata/form (empty hand or weapon) is more than sufficient. If it's a Japanese Jujutsu class, then one technique against an empty hand attack and one against a weapon is probably sufficient. Perhaps also one against a grab or choke.

When I studied Jujutsu, each class involved a technique against a punch, a technique against a kick, a technique against a grab or choke or hold, a technique against a baseball bat, a technique against a knife, and a technique against a gun. That's just too much for one class. It would have been better to focus on one or two, or maybe three, techniques.

If you're taking Aikido, two or three throws are enough. Much more than that becomes difficult to remember.

Tip #10:
Take Advantage
of the Wisdom
and
Generosity of Your More Senior
Fellow Martial Arts Students

Make sure you find more senior students to learn from. Some might be willing to stick around after class, or to meet outside of class, to go over techniques with you. You can gain a tremendous amount of wisdom, insight, and experience from your senior students. Take advantage of this.

If you can't find any senior students willing to help you out, then you're probably at the wrong school. A good school will have some senior students that are always ready to help and share what they've learned with you. Take advantage of this.

I know that I have been very fortunate in my martial arts training experience, especially with so many black belt and black sash senior students always helping me out as I was progressing in rank when I was a novice in whatever system I was studying at the time. Some of the advice I have been sharing with you in these booklets comes from their wisdom and experience, and some comes from their insights after they learned from making mistakes. Their wisdom can often be priceless.

Tip #11:
Do Not Practice Sloppily,
Rather Always
Practice Correctly

This is especially a problem with solo practice, with kata or forms training, and with weapons training. If you have a time constraint, or space constraint, you might be tempted to practice in a half-ass sort of way.

Rather than aid your practice, what this does is provide you with repetition of poorly executed techniques. Instead of helping you practice well, it rather instills bad skills and hardwires errors into your muscle memory. You don't want to do this!

If you don't have time to practice everything (I promise you won't, especially as you progress), then don't. Just focus on what's most important or on what's doable in light of the time constraints. This is a real problem for me.

Although I no longer train in all of the styles I've studied, I actively practice Aikido, Chi Kung, Hsing-I, Karate, Kung Fu, Pa Kua, and Tai Chi. How do I find the time for this? It's not easy. I can't spend equal time on each.

Even if I were just doing one style it would be difficult. If I only practiced Aikido, I'd have to find time to go to the dojo and practice the techniques and taking falls, as well as using the Jo staff, and also the bokken wooden sword. If all I did was Kung Fu, I'd have to find time for practicing the hand techniques, the kicks, the empty hand forms, as well as the weapons. That's a lot of practice!

But I practice all of these each week, not every day. You have to organize your own schedule in such a way that you have time to practice, but always practice well. If you don't have room, say, for practicing a weapon, then don't practice it.

Better to practice it well empty hand as if you had the weapon (easier to do with a Japanese sword or with a knife, than with a spear), or don't practice it at all, than to practice it poorly.

Tip #12:
Be Creative
in Finding Additional Ways
to Practice/Exercise
Throughout the Day

I will be highly beneficial for you if you can bring in practicing at odd moments throughout your day. I'll talk much more about this in future blogposts as well as in a future booklet, but you need to learn to use your odd moments to practice martial arts or gain conditioning.

What are some examples? Let's start with conditioning. I'll provide a few examples of both conditioning and practice, and hopefully that will spark your imagination so you'll be able to apply this to yourself and your own training needs and goals:

1) Take the stairs whenever possible. This is an example often found in books on how to lose weight. But for our purposes, burning calories is not as important—unless that's one of your goals for martial arts training—but taking the stairs has many other benefits. It strengthens glutes, thighs, and calves. It also helps with balance. It can also aid your cardio training, especially if you try to take the stairs briskly, or even jog them. Finally, it can help with your training to be more aware of your surroundings, if you incorporate observation training into your martial arts practice and day-to-day life. Taking the stairs might not always be safe, depending on where you are, but take them whenever you can.

2) When you have to wait, on the phone, or at the dentist, try to visualize your techniques.

3) Practice various stance and power techniques at intervals when you can. Examples, for different martial arts styles: sit in seiza (on your knees, as in Aikido practice) alternating between "live" toes and flat toes, while watching a movie at home, or while using the computer. Walk along the hallways in your house in the various stances your style uses. If you work on power training using your inner hip and by digging your feet in the ground (techniques that are broadly applicable to the martial arts), practice this when standing in line at the store, or in your office. Do some of your reading or television/movie watching in various stances.

4) Hang a piece of paper at face level near your desk where you work, and strike it with finger jabs, or other strikes appropriate to your style, throughout the day as you work.

5) Install a makiwara on your car dashboard to punch and strike while you sit in traffic—Bruce Lee was famous for doing this.

6) Walk around the house with a hollow bamboo stalk to gently beat your body with (shins, thighs, chest, ribs, back, arms, forearms) as you move from room to room, or else use your own hands to do the same.

7) Do some light stretches as soon as you get out of bed in the morning, and before going to bed at night.

8) Install a pull-up bar in a door frame of your home, and, if you can't do many pull-ups, use it on certain days of the week when entering or exiting the room.

9) Walk to where you are going as much as possible.

10) Start imagining the people around you could attack you—so long as this doesn't get dangerous—and imagine what you would do in various circumstances. Start watching where people have their hands as you walk around. Are their hands in their pockets, behind their backs, etc. If they were going to attack you with a weapon, where might they place their hands in order to gain access to a weapon.

11) If you have sufficient space, and it's not a danger with kids around or others, keep different practice weapons in different rooms of your home where there's sufficient space to practice them, and then practice a technique with them there, so long as there really is sufficient space. This is advice I have followed regularly, except the part about sufficient space—and I've suffered a lot because of it. So, be careful and use common sense.

Tip #13:
Practice
Even When Travelling

Only take breaks from practice when you are sick or injured, or you just can't because of the circumstances. But don't let travelling for business or pleasure be an excuse not to practice.

It's not safe these days to travel even with practice weapons usually, but if you're staying at a hotel (or someone's house), you can usually find a broom. That broom can become a Jo staff, a very short Bo or long staff (for a form), a very long short staff (Filipino style), a wooden sword of any type (Japanese sword, Chinese straight sword, Chinese broadsword, etc.).

Use your imagination, but try to stick to the rules of however whatever weapon you're imagining it to be. In addition to this, most hotels provide workout rooms, many provide pools, and some even provide running tracks. There's often room for kata/forms practice where there are running tracks.

Again, take the stairs. Walk wherever you can. I've practiced forms/kata (even using broomsticks) in hotel rooms all over the globe. You can also do bodyweight exercises no matter how cramped the space. Be creative, but don't let travel get in the way of your martial arts practice.

Even if you're an Aikido practitioner and can't practice with a partner, and don't want or can't pay a mat fee at a local dojo, or just can't squeeze it into your schedule, you can still practice with a broom as a wooden sword (bokken) or as a Jo staff. You can still perform the rowing exercise and other warm ups. You can practice the basic back roll on your hotel bed. Don't give up, and be creative!

Tip #14:
How to Rest Effectively

Let's face it, your body needs rest. Your body can probably afford to lightly stretch every day and perhaps run through a few techniques each day as well. If you're practicing an internal Chinese martial art, like Chi Kung or Tai Chi, your body can take that every day as well. But in general, it's good to rest your body. Your muscles only grow as you sleep. This is why Bodybuilders take "cat naps" throughout the day. So, make sure you get enough sleep each night, or as much you can. Take a nap whenever the opportunity avails itself, even if it's just a 5 minute power nap, or even if you just have to lay down and close your eyes. Your body needs rest to grow and perform at it's best.

A final word. A number of my readers have been following my blog, Pat Smith Martial Arts, patsmithmartialarts.wordpress.com. and that's a good place to find out more tips about the martial arts, and also about my future writing projects. These initial booklets on *Essential Tips for Beginning Martial Artists* are general in nature, and can apply to whatever martial arts style you study. On my blog, I likewise include general information on the martial arts, but I also include posts devoted to specific styles that I'm familiar with, like Aikido and Kung Fu. I plan on writing articles, booklets, and books on these topics as well in the future.

Please check out my martial arts blog, Pat Smith Martial Arts, at patsmithmartialarts.wordpress.com for more information on the martial arts and my new writing projects

About the Author:

Pat Smith has nearly thirty years' experience in the martial arts. He studied a variety of martial arts styles including Chinese, Japanese, Korean, and American styles.

Pat's broadest experience is in the Chinese styles. He studied a variety of the internal styles of Chinese martial arts that aid health and well-being as well prove to be quite devastating in combat: Chi Kung, Hsing-I Chuan, Pa Kua Chang, and Tai Chi Chuan. He also studied a number of different Kung Fu styles: Monkey style, various Northern Praying Mantis styles, Northern Shaolin, Sun Pin, and Wing Chun. His Chinese training included weapons training. In addition, he studied the Chinese grappling arts of Chin-Na and Shuai Jiao.

His experience in the Korean arts includes Tang Soo Do and Tae Kwon Do. The majority of his training in Japanese styles has been in Aikido and Aikijujutsu.

His primary American training is in a rare synthetic Karate style from the Midwest which resembles a combination of Mixed Martial Arts and Israeli Krav Maga, a style tailor made for vicious street self-defense as well as for military and security hand-to-hand combat. Pat has taught Aikijujutsu, Chin-Na, Hsing-I, Kung Fu, the exclusive American synthetic style, and other arts, to select private students. Pat also hosts a martial arts blog, Pat Smith Martial Arts, patsmithmartialarts.wordpress.com. And be sure to check out my Facebook page. You can also follow me on Twitter @PatSmithMartial.

If you enjoyed this booklet, or my other e-booklet of tips, *Essential Tips for Beginning Martial Artists*, then be sure to check out my new electronic resource on using palm sticks (like kubotans) for self-defense from Amazon.com.

Palm Stick Self-Defense Guide:
What to Look for in this Devastating &
Practical Defense Tool

As well as my new introductory text on Kung Fu:

Secrets of Kung Fu Mastery: The
Fundamentals

And

Essential Self-Defense Tips